The Flower Codes
Plant Spirit Teachings for your Soul to Blossom.

Heidi Wedd

With herbal introductions by Pamela Scott

Copyright © Heidi Wedd & Pamela Scott, 2024

All rights reserved. This book or any portion thereof may not be reproduced or used in any manner whatsoever without the express written permission of the authors.

Published by The Flower Spring

ISBN: 978-1-7635424-0-2 paperback
ISBN: 978-1-7635424-1-9 ebook

Photographs © Heidi Wedd
Botanical illustrations © Jonathan Beresford
Cover design by Nina Saile

Disclaimer: The information in this book is not intended to be used as a substitute for medical advice. Anyone with a medical condition should seek a qualified practitioner.

Table of Contents

Preface **5**
   My Journey: Herbs, Plant speak and Flowers 5
   Remembering the Flowers.. 9

The Flower Codes.. **11**
   The Flower Codes Pathway 13
   Working with The Flower Codes 14
   The Flower Code Essences... 14
   How to take. 15

The Flower Portals **16**
   The Sacred Birth Portal 16

Feverfew.. **18**
   Names & Etymology 19
   Herbal Introduction 19
   Feverfew Flower Code 21

Borage or Starflower... **29**
   Names & Etymology 30
   Herbal Introduction 30
   Borage Flower Code 32

Cherry Blossom... **38**
   Names & Etymology: 39
   Herbal Introduction 39
   Cherry Blossom Flower Code 40

Postscript: Sacred Birth, Sacred Earth....................**45**
Resources **46**
About the Authors **47**

Preface

My Journey: Herbs, Plant speak and Flowers

It was in the midst of my own dark night of the soul in my early 20s that I discovered herbs at a deeper level. I still recall the tangible moment of "rock bottom" that had been coming for some time. And while I wasn't to know it then, that moment marked a significant turning point, a crossroads in my life that only now, I am eternally grateful for, as it very gently led me towards a pathway of healing, growth and the rich world of flowers and herbs.

It still amazes me now, how the herbs found me. I stumbled across a small herbal store called The Hierophant that had a herbal course about to begin. My heart sang as I looked at the program. I had never been so clear about anything before.

Kim Dudley, a visionary herbalist and acupuncturist was to become a new mentor. Every week, a group of us gathered in the small bookstore to learn about one herb in depth. Not just its actions and constituents, but its essential nature. Kim, an early student of Dorothy Hall, had taken her work of herbal person pictures to another level. Combined with his wisdom as an acupuncturist, nurse, the nature of homeopathy, Jungian theory, shamanism, alchemical spagyrics and meditation; without knowing it, we had all signed up to a life changing adventure! For each herb, we learned of its use in history and folklore, its medicinal uses and what Kim termed its Primary disease and emotional theme. For each herb, there was a corresponding disease process and a specific emotional pattern (doubt, resentment, pride, etc.) that would tend to manifest in various physical areas or imbalances, which he termed secondary actions. Each herbal plant family he had corresponded to an acupuncture point. The largest plant family, the Asteraceae for example, corresponds to Colon 4 - one of the most major points in acupuncture that can tend a broad range of imbalances.

Our herbal community connected well as we practiced on ourselves, family and friends and experienced amazing responses - all using doses of less than 5 drops of tincture. The deeper you know a herb at its core, the less you need! In the first class, I sat next to a woman called Pam and we have been friends ever since - bonded by herbs, years of study together and a parallel evolving in the ways of the world. I'm so grateful to have her write the herbal introduction, though it does little to express her wealth of knowledge that extends much further than is within these pages.

Parallel to the herb course, I studied with Kim's business partner, Tim Thomas who taught us homeopathy with plenty of Welsh hilarity and remarkably lifelike examples of each remedy. We began with simple first aid, and slowly expanded until we were experiencing deep insights on the minerals, plants and animals of homeopathy with him. Amidst our herbal studies, we were required to practice spagyric herbal medicine making, guided by Kim and Tim. This was an incredible lived experience of a herb that is hard to forget.

After this three-year life changing journey, many students went on to study with Dorothy Hall in order to get their 'qualification'. I chose to get my 'official paper' through homeopathy and studied with Isaac Golden for the next few years. For my final assignment I conducted a homeopathic proving of a butterfly. This would be all-consuming for over a year as I lived out, documented and eventually published this transformative proving. (Blue Triangle Butterfly: A Homeopathic Proving, 2005.)

A proving is when you gather a group of people to consume a substance and then meticulously document the physical, mental, emotional and spiritual symptoms the substance creates in them. Homeopathy, based on the premise of 'like cures like' and with well over 200 years of experience to support its efficacy, is quite scientific in this manner. We know what a substance treats by what it has caused in a healthy person. In a proving, each participant is supervised, and symptoms assessed for relevancy daily. Conducting this proving was another turning point for me. Having been in the heady learning of hundreds of homeopathic remedies in my studies, this was the experiential wisdom that I was craving. While I was not taking the butterfly remedy myself (no harm done to the butterfly by the way), I lived out the experience through all the participants and my own life that year, which went through incredible change.

After this, I knew I wanted more direct, experienced wisdom in my plant realm again, more spagyric making, more 'provings' and more plant communication. So I set out to learn more. Back then, there was little around on plant communication, so I set off for Findhorn in Scotland to learn from Dorothy Maclean - a cofounder of this incredible ecovillage. It was she who had begun to receive communications from the plants, and which along with the other cofounders, had implemented the insights received. After a few years, scientists were visiting their community and remarking at the 'impossibility' of such large vegetables and plants growing on such barren sandy soil in a harsh cold climate. Nothing is impossible when you're cocreating with the plant devas[1] though!!

I returned to Australia and practiced plant communication as much as I could. It helped me. I grounded into the earth more. But I struggled to make time to do it. I began holding courses in plant alchemy and spagyrics - I had been making my own over the years, but the power of circle is exponential when working with plants.

---

[1] Deva – the unique soul blueprint and personality of the plant, what is commonly called *plant spirit,* though in an alchemical context it is the *plant soul.*

Eventually, I decided to walk the Bibbulmun track solo - a 1000km walking track in Western Australia, with the intention of deepening my connection with nature, of spending much more time communicating with the plants without the distractions of daily life and people. While it wasn't quite the 'quiet' time I was expecting, I did find a deeper connection, though not in the way I had thought. You can read about this adventure in the book (Wild Flower Walker: A Pilgrimage to Nature on the Bibbulmun Track).

After this journey, my life took a wild tangent as I went back to university to become a midwife - an experience I try to remember as little as possible! Being a midwife is very special. Working in a hospital system I found trying at the best of times. In my second year of study, I received a very strong dream and woke with a calling to live in Alice Springs. So when I finished my degree, I became a graduate midwife there. It still amazes me how spirit works. I applied nowhere else. There were hundreds of applicants, and yet the whole time, I knew I would be one. Four of us were accepted at Alice and I moved there shortly after. The land had a strong effect on me. Being in daily contact with indigenous women who were deeply connected to land was equally transforming. I soaked it in. I loved it out there. And I struggled.

Somewhere through the year, I came into contact with my next teacher, Kim Leyland, who was offering a small course in nature shamanism. This rocked my world! Shamanic journeying was a new way into the plant realm that felt so deep and easy. I took every chance I had to learn from the nature beings in my spare time.

And this is where my current journey with the flower codes began. The more I dived into the plant realm, the more I received the message that I needed to connect with my ancestors. I didn't want to, that sounded boring and I had no idea what it meant. This was before ancestral healing became a fad. But the message was persistent and when Kim happened to mention an ancestral course that was about to happen with Mary Shutan, I decided it was time. Now I look back and see how crucial it was. It took me some years to develop these ancestral relationships and to dive into healing work with them. Ancestral exploration, along with a potent vision quest as part of a training with Jane Hardwicke Collings (another teacher whose work on cycles and birth imprints has been invaluable to my journey) led to discovering latent gifts within my ancient lineage ready to awaken.

Remembering the Flowers...

One of these gifts has been The Flower Codes. The flower codes were an inner journey for several years before bringing them even into conversation with people.

Each flower came to me of its own accord, and I dived into learning about its 'code' (their own terminology, not mine) for a period of time - often several months. I journeyed and communed with the plant repeatedly until they let me know they were complete and the next flower code appeared. The physical flower code essences were made only when the inner work was at a certain level and the flower devas gave the go ahead. The pieces came gradually, and what I share in this book is a growing body of knowledge. Codes that can be awakened in all of us.

Activating this wisdom within myself took a lot of time, energy and personal work, along with personal life changes that I needed to make along the way. Some requests took me months to fulfill! It has, and continues to be a journey of commitment, that is filled with joy and its fair share of challenges!

Fast forward a number of years and I began to share the flower code teachings along with plant communication basics in circle. This became the Shamanic Herbalism pathways, which evolved over the years into the Flower Codes Training. Working in this way brought a whole other level of activation both personally (each time a slightly different spiral of the flowers teachings unfold), but more excitingly, in the collective. Witnessing the awesome shifts occurring in the people called to the flower pathways has been incredibly gratifying, but even more is to see how their inner flowering effects those around them. Like pollen that spreads through the air, the slow, subtle and gentle shifts in the collective, have surprised me. It appears it really is the subtle changes that are the most profoundly transformative. The butterfly effect in motion.

The Flower Codes

Every flower has a unique vibration or code; a teaching; an essence that it carries through its whole being. To tune into the depths of a plant is to understand this message.

When you meet a person for the first time, you learn a little about them – maybe their name, where they're from etc. Even should you have a deeply intimate conversation with them, there's only so much you can know at one meeting. Plants are the same. Relationships with them take time. Information comes out in layers. Even how easily they connect is unique to each plant, just like with people. Herbs are a great place to begin the cocreation journey with, as people have had conversations with them for centuries. The relationship has already been cultivated, though there is always more to learn. Plants evolve alongside humanity. If we go purely by old knowledge, we will miss much of their relevance and healing gifts in the now. This is one reason developing skills of deep listening and direct, embodied wisdom of a plant is so important. With herbs, there is already a paved pathway to communion, making the process easier. On the other hand, there are plants in the bush that feel as if talking to humans is so far in their distant memories, they've forgotten how to commune with us as much as humanity as a collective has with them.

Making herbal alchemical spagyrics is a great way to deepen with a plant as you are working in depth and sharing a transformative process with the plant. What I have found after countless alchemical adventures with different plants within groups, is that at a certain point in the alchemy, the information becomes collective. Generally (there are always exceptions to the rule), plants will share bits and pieces. Different people obviously pick up different information and themes begin to emerge. This continues as the layers of the plant emerge and are shared via communicating with it and experiencing the process through the alchemical vessel that is the group field. At some point, the themes begin to coalesce and everything begins to make sense. This is when you get to the core or soul of the plant, it's essential nature or essence, its unique teaching. Once you understand this, all the myriad different symptoms, insights and actions (periphery) begin to make sense as you have touched its core essence and can see *why* it works in that way. See diagram. In this series, I am focusing on sharing the themes within the core essence.

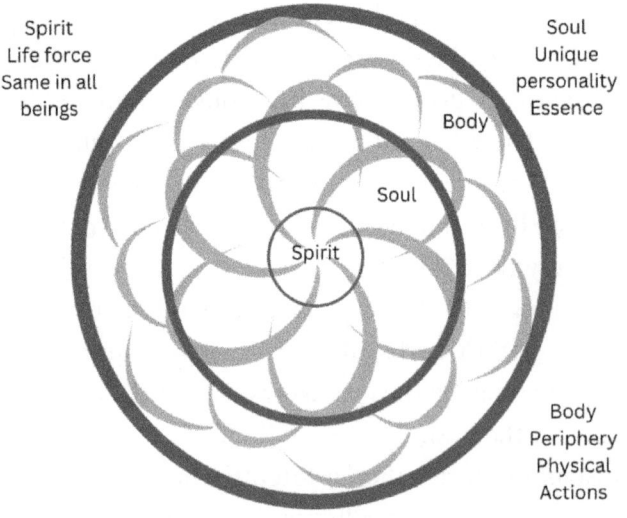

When I began working with the flower codes (as they called themselves), they spoke to me of awakening our DNA. At the time, I had no understanding of what this actually meant, though now it is common in our language. They also shared with me that in times long before ours, this information was much more accessible. By simply smelling a flower, its "code" would be awakened within us. We would open up to an understanding or way of being that this flower was keeper of. While this knowledge was slowly forgotten over time, remnants remain within us. Throughout history, there have always been those who held herbal lore and wisdom and the ability to unlock a code and activate it in another - sometimes simply by placing the flower in their psychic field.

While we are not quite back at that state of being, the flower codes are coming back into consciousness now for a reason – because we are ready to come back to that state of awareness again. That is the intention of these particular flowers and their codes – to reawaken and help us remember this way of being.

Flowers *were* and *are* a language. Each has a unique vibration.

The flower codes activate specific states of being within us. They are like archetypal energies, simple and divine. Activating and awakening these natural states of being within ourselves, reawakens them on the Earth. By journeying with the flowers, we can begin to embody a Sacred Earth consciousness.

The Flower Codes Pathway

To this point in time (it is an ever-growing body of learning), there are nine central flower codes. These are about awakening a Sacred Earth consciousness within ourselves. They form a pathway of awakening through the language of flowers.

In all truly holistic healing, we heal from the centre out, focusing not on symptoms but on deep cause. With the flower codes we do the same - we begin by activating our true and natural state – our unique essence. The pathway of the flower codes takes us along this in a step by step manner, gently yet surely.

As we move along the pathway of the portal flowers and touch the natural states, it will likely trigger the need for some of the ally flowers such as the healing herb flowers. As we see the transgression away from our natural state, the wounds arise and the need for healing may appear. As an example, within the first three flowers, we are remembering birth as a sacred portal, the blueprint of its highest vibration as an initiation and gateway into the physical realm. However, an enormous percentage of people on the planet have not experienced birth in this way, instead experiencing interruption or trauma. While the core flowers help us to remember and clear, there are times when we may need to use healing herb flowers to clear the trauma and wounding – Calendula, Bellis, Hypericum, Yarrow are a few examples. Working firstly with the core flowers, yet calling in the others as needed, we begin to reweave our DNA, the earthly strands we are embedded within, along with the Earth itself.

Working with The Flower Codes

There are a myriad of ways to awaken the flower code teachings within us. Conscious work with the themes below along with immersing yourself in the field of the flower is all that is required.

The Flower Code essences are an easy way in. For a deeper and wholistic immersion you can join the Flower Codes Training, in which we develop communications with the plant and work with their teachings in order to fully activate and embody them within us.

The Flower Code Essences

The flower codes are similar yet different to flower essences. While they are completely safe and can be taken in the same way as flower essences, their action and intention are slightly different. They work to activate and remember states of consciousness within us and contain a cocreated and *evolved* form of the flower. Because they have been 'evolved' through the co-creative process with the flower, some of the work is already done for you. However, it is always better to work consciously alongside the plant. This enables deeper healing and a recognition of the inner processes involved.

Each flower code is made using specific instructions which differ with each flower. Some are pure flower essences activated with sound; others are a combination of spagyrics, flower essences and homeopathic potencies blended over a certain period of time, at a specific time of the year, with sound, intention and devic activation. They are made when the devas say the time is ready, so not all have been made to this point in time.

How to take.

The general suggestion is to take the drops 2-3 times a day over a 3-5 week period. However, this should be tempered with your own knowing and feeling. Take as needed and if you feel to stop, stop. Come back when you are ready.

Before you start, set an intention or journal around why you have chosen this essence. Then over the weeks you are taking it, check in and journal regularly as to what is arising, and shifting in you. Engage in the process for a more potent shift in the activation process. Use your intuition and inner knowing. Maybe a flower has called you or has shown up in your life. Trust that and start there. If in doubt, start with the portal flowers – Feverfew is the beginning of the pathway.

The supporting flower code groups are allies to assist with what arises when working with the core flowers. There is a reason they are common herbs found around the world – most people can benefit from them!

The Flower Portals

There are nine core flower codes or portals. Each of these is a gateway into a whole realm that contains a world in itself.

What was slowly revealed to me in connecting with them, was that these nine flowers are the original codes of a Sacred Earth reality and form a pathway to remembering our ancient Lemurian consciousness. The best I can explain this state of being from the glimpses I have experienced is a world in which everything (plants, animals, mountains, lakes, elementals etc.) is considered sacred, where every action takes into account the whole because the effect is felt immediately throughout oneself. Separation is an illusion we currently exist in. In this connected space, each unique flower can be felt and experienced directly and immediately.

These core flower codes or portals support us to remember and reawaken this way of being that has been held dormant within our DNA for aeons.

The Sacred Birth Portal

The Sacred Birth Portal contains the first three of the core flower codes – each a gateway within itself. They work powerfully as a trio as well as individually.

The flower codes of the Sacred Birth Portal activate our inner sacred birth pathways. Like a prayer for all births to be sacred, they help us to *know* what sacred birth feels like so that we can create that for ourselves and others. They activate our divine blueprint for birthing, helping us to remember our birth right – that every birth (be it your own, birthing a creative project into the world, or birthing a babe into your arms) is a sacred portal to the divine.

While we will go into each one separately, the three together nurtures our ability to:
- *create sacred space, prepare the sacred vessel.*
- *remember and allow our soulstar self to birth into the world with a courageous push;*
- *joyfully and softly integrate into the body or material realm, receiving and nurturing ourselves into being.*

Together they cover the literal phases of birth as well as the metaphorical.

Feverfew

Sacred Space

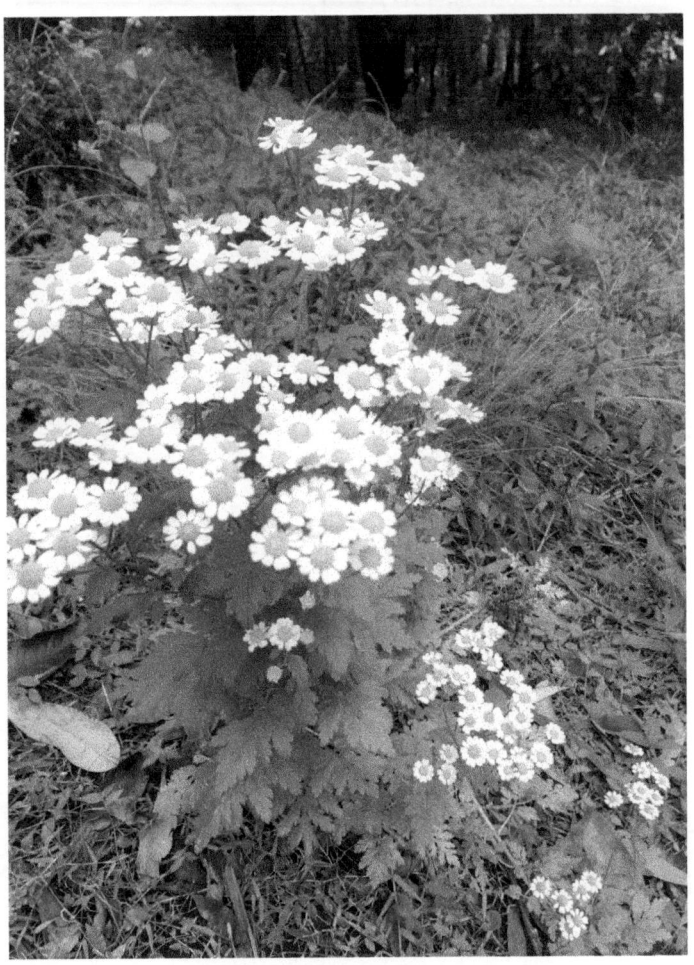

Tanacetum Parthenium
Asteraceae

Names & Etymology

Bachelors Buttons, Featherfew, Febrifuge, Flirtweed, Flirtwort, Bride's buttons, Maids weed, Devils daisy, Featherfoil, Santa Maria, Mother Herb, Mutterkraut, Matricaria, Partenelle.

Chrysanthemum parthenium.

Tanacetum comes from *athanatos* meaning *immortal*. Thanatos is the Greek god of death.

Parthenium derives from the Greek *Parthenos* which means *virgin* or *maid*.

Matricaria derives from *matrix* meaning *womb*.

Pyrethrum from Greek *pur* pyro = fire referring to the fiery taste of the root.

Herbal Introduction

By Pam Scott

Feverfew is originally native to the Balkans, has a daisy-like flower and is unusual in that it deters insects and bees. Perfect for planting around vegetable gardens and houses to keep pests away, herbalists of old would plant Feverfew around their garden to purify the air. It can be used in open weave bags in the closet to repel moths. It is a tough perennial that happily self-seeds in most soils and benefits from a prune back occasionally.

Feverfew was traditionally considered more of a women's herb hence its name 'Parthenium' (Greek: *girl/virgin*). It was used to open and increase the flow of the menses, expel the placenta and cleanse the uterus. It is often included in herb blends for vaginal steaming preparations to 'clean and purify'.

Its popularity goes back 2000 years when Dioscorides prescribed it for childbirth and to reduce fevers. Culpeper, in the 1600s, also valued it for 'strengthening the womb' and to increase menstrual flow, even more specifically for 'hysteria' or angry outbursts in relation to the flow of the menses. He also prescribed it for headache and migraine relief. This pain relief is what Feverfew is most known for. The parthenolide component of the plant has been found to inhibit prostaglandins which may be responsible for migraines. Its vasodilating properties may be helpful here too if blood flow needs regulating.

Eating 2 leaves a day can reduce the frequency and severity of headaches. Although very bitter, they can be mixed with other foods to disguise the taste and though unpleasant, this bitterness is helpful in increasing bile flow, stimulating digestion and appetite.

Feverfew's ability to block prostaglandins and histamines and decrease inflammatory conditions in the body makes it perfect for hot arthritic conditions and allergic reactions. The crushed leaves can bring relief rubbed on to insect bites or as a mosquito repellent. Cherokees would soak tired swollen feet in a Feverfew foot bath.

Many of Feverfew's actions allow the opening, release and movement of conditions that could be classed as stagnant, cramped, constricted and congested. This can also apply to a 'stuck' mental state where there is no movement. Feverfew creates a safe place to allow opening and releasing on all levels.

Flowers are best harvested just as they are about to bloom and leaves can be harvested at any time. They can be frozen to ensure a plentiful supply is at hand.

Sensitivity to Feverfew can display in mouth ulcers, throat irritation or gastrointestinal upsets. Check your sensitivity by rubbing a leaf on your wrist and seeing if a rash develops within 24 hours.

As it is a uterine stimulant, large amounts are contraindicated in pregnancy and lactation. It is best avoided if taking blood thinning medications.

Actions - Vasodilator, diaphoretic, anti-inflammatory, decongestant, antihistamine, bitter digestive, anti-cramping, relaxing and also a stimulant, analgesic, tonic, antidepressant, carminative and emmenagogue.

Feverfew Flower Code

Feverfew is the first of the nine portal flower codes. It marks both the beginning and the ending and as such, energetically relates to Winter Solstice and New Moon - the deep inward time in which the transition from dark to light occurs. As the first of the Sacred Birth trio, it holds an essential role in creating a safe space for the magic of creation to unfold. In a sense it is a herb of the void from which new life begins to take root in the darkness deep below. It covers conception and the inner gestation of life.

The essence or core teaching of Feverfew is the creation and protection of *Sacred Space*.

Sacred Space - the Alembic or Sacred Vessel

In alchemy, the *alembic* is the sacred alchemical vessel, a sealed container in which the transformations take place. Fire is one of the key alchemical processes that burns away what is no longer needed in order to reveal the gold that lies within.

Sacred Space is a key part of ceremony, ritual and spiritual practice. It can be as simple as lighting a candle and allowing the mind to fall into silence until all that exists is the present moment. Or it may be the elaborate church rituals of swinging gigantic incense burners. Even churches themselves are buildings that set up sacred space by their very architecture. We can see it in the smoking ceremonies of various indigenous cultures and in different yet essentially similar ways around the world. In fact, many ancient indigenous cultures *lived* in a continuous state of sacred space and Feverfew can help us start to reawaken this, so that we can return to this natural state of being.

Essentially setting up sacred space is to provide a safe container from which the divine can enter, transform, communicate and create. When we set up sacred space, we are stepping into a zone in which we know something greater than ourselves is at play. Within, is an acknowledgement that we are not in full control. Our part is to ensure we have cleansed, cleared, purified and set up a clear, protective container, so that the magic can unfold within. Intention is another key to sacred space – becoming clear on the why helps direct the process, and in effect places boundaries around what occurs.

Feverfew and Sacred Space
Feverfew holds the flower coding of creating a safe, sacred space. To make friends and learn from Feverfew will awaken this ability within you.

It is a herb to activate through potent threshold times such as birth and death. Or any of the myriad transition times in life that involve an ending and a new beginning and the liminal space in between. It is at these times that vulnerability is high and a great need for protection is necessary so that the transition can unfold gracefully. Feverfew plays a key role in creating a ring of protection in which we can relax and flow with the changes knowing we are safe.

Fever-FEW

As a fumigator, Feverfew has a centrifugal action that repels the negative or harmful energies that create illness. Well known to prevent and clear fevers, the Feverfew deva shares that the way it does this is by throwing off the pathogens or negative influences that *evoke* the fever response within the body. Fever is simply the body's natural way of burning up unwanted substances or energies. Once the cause of the fever has been released, the need for a fever is removed. Feverfew treats a fever at the root cause, not by lowering the body's temperature, but by clearing the *cause* of the rise in temperature.

An activated Feverfew within us, maintains a sacred space clear of harmful influences. It protects by warding off negative energy so that we can stay open, relaxed and expansive knowing we are safe. It is to have a ring of protection around us, within which we can breathe and expand into.

Winter Solstice, New Moon, the dark night of the Soul, the Void.

Feverfew is particularly related to the New Moon or Winter Solstice - the longest night or the darkest times in our lives. After the longest night, there is a movement outwards towards the periphery again. We slowly start to open up and expand as the daily light begins to grow in length. Feverfew relates to the periphery, and just as it has a centrifugal action, it helps us to expand fully into ourselves after the deepest contraction of Winter or a personal dark night of the soul.

Winter marks the time when the roots are growing deep below the surface of the earth, when growth is happening in the unseen realms, just as a fetus grows invisibly in the dark watery realms of the womb. Feverfew covers this pre-birth period - from void to conception in the womb, all throughout pregnancy and right through the first stages of labour. It relates to the phase from

Winter solstice (when energies are growing deep within the waters of the womb) to just before Imbolc when the sprouts are ready to break through to the surface of the earth and birth into the light.

The Alembic of the body - the Womb.

We have looked at Feverfew as the creator of Sacred Space, so it is not hard to see the relationship it has to the womb - the alembic or alchemical vessel within a woman's body, which holds space for the transformation of creation to unfold.

Feverfew used to be known as *Matricaria parthenium* from the Latin *matrix* meaning *womb,* and the womb was often known as the *Mother* in old times. As Culpeper states, Feverfew *"...is a general strengthener of the womb and to remedy such infirmities as a careless midwife has there caused. It cleanses the womb, expels the afterbirth and does a woman all the good she can desire of a herb. It is chiefly used for the disease of the mother..."*

On a larger level, Feverfew is a little like the cosmic womb of creation, the vessel that holds us all. The void from which all begins...

The Midwife's Herb - Protector of Thresholds and Guardian of Incarnation.

As guardian of the gates of incarnation, and also to those who are leaving the body at the end of life, the spirit of Feverfew is like a protective circle of birth/death midwives that call a babe forth from the womb into the birthing tunnel, and that also watch over the transition from life into the spirit world again. On another level, it is the circle of ancestral grandmothers that call forth the spirit to incarnate in the world, planting a soul seed into fertile ground for the soul to sprout.

Just as Culpeper noted - if you don't have a good midwife or a healthy Feverfew, then you're going to need Feverfew! A holistic, conscious midwife or birth keeper is Feverfew incarnated in human form. Their role in the early and first stages of labour is to maintain a sacred space, hold presence, and protect any harmful influences from entering so that the woman birthing can fully relax and journey to the stars to bring her baby to earth. A midwife knows how to 'sit on her hands' and avoid interfering or 'doing for' as a vital part of maintaining the sacredness of birth. While she appears to be doing nothing, her presence is vital to maintain safety, protect the space, and help 'call forth' the incarnating being for she knows the birth/death threshold like the back of her hand.

When this external ring of protection and sacred space is maintained, both the birthing woman and her babe can expand into the space allowing the sacred magic of birth to unfold.

Feverfew is the guardian that watches over incarnation. It calls forth the soul to be planted in the soil of life and to take root and grow. In this sense it is a herb of grounding and earthing, of coming into being and incarnating into the earthly realm. Many experience the Feverfew flower code as deeply grounding.

Fertility

Feverfew is a great flower code to engage with when trying to conceive - to clear the way energetically and physically for a babe to incarnate. Several people have become pregnant while taking the Feverfew flower code – some called to work deeply with obstacles that are in the way of a fertile soil. Feverfew can work to clear the womb of influences that may be preventing conception, and create a sacred nourishing womb that is ripe for the picking.

Perimenopause

Menopause is known as the great 'change of life' and Feverfew can be a potent ally in navigating this transition. As always, it helps to clear space so that the new phase of life over the threshold can unfold. The cessation of bleeding can be accompanied by hot flushes – the body's 'fever' to burn off what is no longer required. What was once released through the monthly blood, now must find a new way of being processed, and hot flushes may be one of the ways it deals with the buildup of influences. Flushes are a mini fever and Feverfew can work with them in the same way. The alchemical process of burning all that is no longer valid is an apt analogy, especially as the source of them lies within the transitioning womb. Flushes can also be the result of the hypothalamus attempting to over-control a system that is not responding hormonally the way it used to. Perimenopause can see the hormones fluctuating wildly as the body find its new hormonal balance. Working energetically to connect your ovaries and the glandular control centre within your head can be helpful. The increase of headaches and migraines in perimenopause can be another indication for Feverfew. Known as a 'miracle herb' for migraines, it can work wonders if taken regularly as a preventative.

Feverfew Flower Code Summary

Feverfew creates a sacred safe space within which to expand. It protects and centrifugally wards off negative energies (including pathogens). An activated Feverfew is especially important for all vulnerable transition times - death, birth, menses, rites of passage, dark nights. Feverfew allows us to stay open in these times, to grow and expand through them rather than contract and close down.

Feverfew flower code is useful to clear and set up sacred space. This can be externally or internally. A few drops sprayed or scattered around the boundary can be used to clear the energy, create or consecrate sacred space.

You may need to work with the energy of Feverfew Flower Code if you:

- have trouble creating space in your life;
- are doing too much and not making enough space for what is really important to you at a soul level;
- are going through a vulnerable transition time;
- are a birth keeper, death doula or guardian of any rite of passage;
- are caught in the energy of contraction in order to protect yourself;
- would like to create more space for the divine in your life.
- Would like to prepare for receiving an incarnating being in the womb.
- Have any of the physical symptoms of Feverfew – it's possibly there is space clearing within to be done.

Physical

Without an activated Feverfew, we can get caught in trying to protect ourselves resulting in the energy of contraction.

Common ways this can present:

- Migraines. Essentially these relate to controlling patterns that are set up in order to protect; control is generally based in an underlying fear, a sense of not being safe. Another layer can relate to us not processing toxins effectively, again, the need for repelling and clearing unwanted substances or energies is the realm of Feverfew.
- PMS. The premenstrual phase can be a vulnerable time. If we don't feel safe or have sufficient space to engage with what is arising, prickliness, irritability and contraction can be autopilot ways that are engaged by the body in order to protect and create space for ourselves. "I need space"; "don't come near me"; irritability; pain, cramping; headaches etc. Your body is talking to you.
- Cramps - an obvious contraction.

- Constriction of blood vessels.
- Fevers – when our periphery/boundary/space/immune system has been invaded, the body's natural response is to burn off the unwanted invaders by increasing temperature.
- Womb - Feverfew is a big womb herb that can be used for many womb imbalances and disease processes to bring the womb back to its essential nature of holding and maintaining space for creation - contracting and relaxing when necessary. It can bring on menses, expel placenta, get labour started (i.e. healthy contraction), but it can also relax the uterus when it is time to relax. Culpeper recommends it as a great yoni steaming herb. Menstrual symptoms.
- Fertility – to clear the space in order to provide a fertile soil and nest for conception.
- Birth – Feverfew is useful in early labour as well as all through first stage.
- Perimenopause – hot flushes (*fever*few), headaches, migraines and to protect the space while women cross the great change of life threshold.

Borage / Starflower

Birth

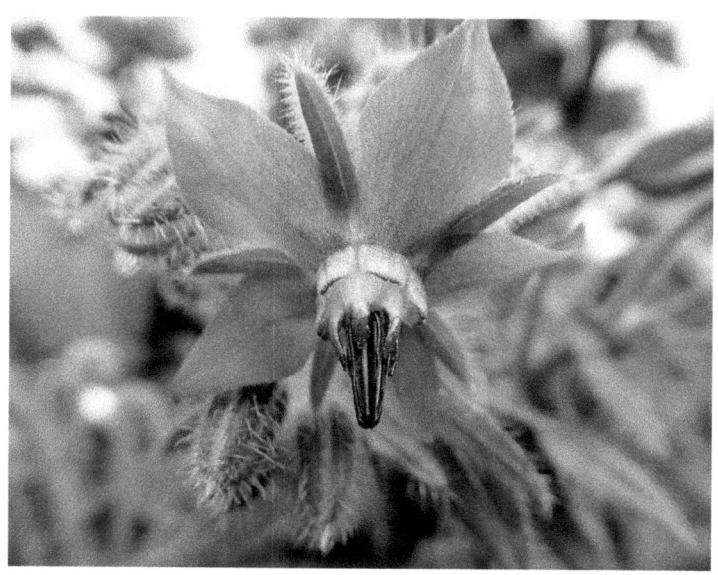

Borago officinalis,

Boraginaceae

Names & Etymology

Borage is also known as Starflower, Bee bread, Bee plant, Cool tankard, Burrage, Bugloss, Corago, Talewort and Ox's Tongue (for its furry leaves).

Borage is thought to be a corruption of *Corago* (*cor* = heart, *ago* = I bring) hence the saying "Borage for Courage."

Burra is Latin for 'hairy garment'

In Celtic it was known as *barrach*, which means *man of courage*. In Welsh is is *Llawenlys*, meaning *herb of gladness*. To the Moors, it was *abourach* = *father of sweat*. Pliny called it *Euphrosinum* as it 'makes man joyful'.

Herbal Introduction

By Pam Scott

Native to the Mediterranean, Borage is a fast-growing perennial that grows to nearly a metre high. It self-seeds very happily in most soils but does not like to be disturbed once growing. It has soft spiny stems and leaves with blue starlike flowers that attract bees. It makes a great honey. The leaves and flowers can be added to salads for their cool cucumber taste.

Borage is a popular companion plant, especially with strawberries. It is said that a strawberry that fruits near Borage will be larger and sweeter than those that don't. Borage also makes a great compost activator.

Borage juice or a poultice of crushed leaves can be put on skin complaints such as ringworm, eczema, acne or hot, dry, itchy rashes. Bathing hot, dry and itchy eyes in a cool infusion is soothing too. This cooling effect aids many inflammatory conditions and a poultice of leaves and flowers is helpful to relieve gout and some painful rheumatic and arthritic symptoms. The diaphoretic action of a cup of tea may help to bring down fevers. A tea of the mucilaginous leaves could help settle dry difficult coughs too.

The seeds are high in GLA (omega 6 fatty acid) and are often sold as Starflower oil to help with skin, menopausal and arthritic complaints. Mixed with Fennel, it increases milk production for nursing mothers.

The flowers and leaves have been steeped into a cordial or wine that was said to lift spirits and gladden hearts.

John Gerard in 1597 said Borage flower syrup 'comforteth the heart, purgeth melancholy and quieteth phrenticke and lunatick person.'

Pliny says 'it maketh a man merry and joyful.'

It was supposedly given to Helen of Troy steeped in wine to lift her spirits and ease her grief with any possible loss of friends or family in battle. 'Thou couldst not grieve or shed a tear for them.' Roman soldiers would drink Borage wine to bring courage and strengthen their spirits before battle.

'I Borage always bring courage'

We now know that Borage revives, nourishes and stimulates the adrenal cortex that produces our fight or flight response and readies the body for stressful or difficult times ahead where we may need courage. It is high in Silica which will give us the grit and determination to carry on. It supports our nervous system, kidneys and heart.

These days we all may need the support of Borage. It's most beneficial where the nervous system is at a point of exhaustion, whether from overwork or prolonged stress. An example could be midlife where we may be exhausted needing to look at a new way of being or phase of life. For whatever is next in life, Borage will nourish, revive and support us. It's a plant that softens, opens up, releases and moves.

There are a couple of cautions with Borage. It shouldn't be taken long term or in large doses as it does have pyrrolizidine alkaloids that may affect the liver and be carcinogenic. The spines on the stems and leaves if handled for too long, may develop a contact dermatitis.

Actions: Febrifuge, diaphoretic, anti-inflammatory, decongestant, diuretic, mucilaginous, galactagogue

Borage Flower Code

Borage is the second of the core flower codes and one of the three Sacred Birth Portal flower teachers. Borage teachings include:

Go Forth
Borage is strong, courageous, and bold. Its movement is forwards. 'Go Forth!' Borage is the energy and the push of Birth.

Birthing new beings or stages into the world requires a significant amount of strength, courage, boldness and the 'push' or 'go forth' energy. Whether it is birthing a child, artistic creations, our true selves or heart projects into the world, all are vulnerable processes that require the sacred space and protection of Feverfew, followed by the courageous forward motion of Borage.

Imbolc
Borage relates to Imbolc - the cross-quarter point on the annual solar cycle that sits midway between Winter solstice and Spring equinox. It marks the first tentative signs of Spring and a subtle shift in the light and length of days. It is said to be when the sprouts breach the surface of the soil and into the light. Like the crescent

three-day young moon that reappears in the sky, Imbolc is the first sign of the light returning after the darkness of Winter. It is the moment of new birth after the wintry, watery darkness of the gestational underworld. Imbolc marks the transition from the watery depths of the collective, into the element of air - ever expanding, growing, light and excitable.

Birth and Cosmic Imprints

Whatever 'baby' you are birthing - be it a child, a creation, a business or a new version of yourself, the phases of birth remain the same. Starflower covers the active second stage of labour - the 'pushing' or 'breathing a baby out' phase, right up until the moment when the babe inhales its first breath.

The second stage of labour generally evokes the urge to activate and engage the process. There is an unmistakeable desire to "push", to move things forward, without force. While the first stage of labour (covered by Feverfew) is dominated by the hormone of oxytocin, the second stage sees a release of adrenalin and the strong, imminent energy of forwards motion that is the signature of Borage. Starflower supports this process by awakening the strength, courage and 'heart' to move through this often intense phase. To cross the threshold. While Feverfew holds space for fertility, conception, gestation and finally the surrendering and opening of the cervix to its full capacity, making way for new life. Borage takes over the reins at transition. Transition is generally marked by overwhelm, 'this is too big', 'I can't cope' are its signature phrases. A threshold is being crossed, a point of no return. This is followed by the second stage of labour – the active phase accompanied by overwhelming urges to push. Pushing is not meant to be forced, but a sensation that happens from within. It is not something that should be directed from outside of you.

The moment of birth is also very significant and a key part of Borage medicine. On one hand, the first inhalation is the breath in which the energies of the cosmos imprint their forces on the babe. The astrological birth chart is a map of these starry imprints – a map of the sky at the moment of birth. This map can be consciously engaged with throughout life to work with our inherent strengths, weaknesses and tendencies.

The experience of birth is also firmly imprinted neurally within a baby. And it is from this experience that a significant number of our imprints of 'what life is' are sourced. These are laid down innately within our brains as complexes of hormones and hormone receptors that unconsciously inform the rest of our lives and the patterns within which we live. Working consciously with our birth imprints to unravel and choose with awareness, the way we live our lives rather than being unconsciously informed by our early programming, is a large part of activating the Starflower gift within ourselves. It is a sad truth, that a high proportion of people alive today, have a significant amount of unresolved birth trauma from the cultural influences of our current birthing systems. The more people that have the courage, strength and tenacity required to face this deep inner birthwork, the more likely it is that the system will change as the culture that continues to support it shifts. The way we birth informs the way we live on the earth. Sacred Birth = Sacred Earth. Violent birth leads to violence on earth.

Cervix - the Gateway.

Starflower has a beautiful plant signature[2] for the cervix - the back of the flower contains a white ring, and the front of the flower with

---

[2] The Doctrine of Signatures is an ancient herbal philosophy that recognises the appearance, growth or properties of a plant can indicate how they affect the human system.

its seeds, appears like a closed cervix. It is the cervix that softens, thins and opens wide in order for birth to occur. It is the opening of the cervix that takes up the majority of time in labour (Feverfew's first stage). And no wonder, for as the cervix opens, so does the heart. It is an opening of love, mostly governed by the unconditional love hormone of oxytocin.

Just as the cervix is the doorway between the inner and outer worlds through which we are born, Starflower is a gateway to the stars - a portal between worlds. It is said that a birthing woman travels to the stars and back during labour to collect her child.

Beyond birth, Starflower can help us travel back to the stars to remember our origins and to reactivate our inner star, just as it can support us to birth into this world.

Star Codes and the Path of the Heart

Star codes, as I understand it from the Starflower deva, are our reason for being, the reason we chose to come to earth. While they are often forgotten at birth, they remain imprinted within our body. In fact, they are stored in *every cell* of our body as light, inactivated as they may be.

Starflower helps us to remember and reactivate our inner light. A light that appears like starlight, but resides within us.

The heart is a key to remembering. When we are on track with our inner light, in resonance with it, the heart smiles. Whenever we listen to the heart and allow it to be an integral part in our decision making, our starlight, which is stored in every cell, starts humming like the bees and shining a little brighter. There is a ripple effect as we begin resonating with our starlight again and this increases the light more, and so on and so forth.

Starflower not only helps us to remember our star path, but brings us the courage to follow the quiet nudges of our soul, the things that make our heart smile and swell with love. Following this path may not always be easy, there will most definitely be challenges and thresholds to cross, but when you listen inwardly, the heart still smiles nonetheless. This is the path to awakening our inner light further. The light that makes us sparkle with delight. Starflower brings the strength to move through our patterning and imprints, so that we can find the starlight within our hearts again. So that we have the courage to *choose* the path of our soul, to remember our starry mission - to shine our light on the earth.

Borage Flower Code is useful for those who give up easily when they reach an obstacle. It can be useful for those who 'go with the flow' a little too much when commitment and conscious action are required. Starflower helps us to do the work that needs to be done and brings the courage to face obstacles and fearful situations "head first". It helps us realise that the only reason we are here is to follow our soul path and that that is how we shine! When we shine our light, others around us are encouraged to open their heart and follow their path to shining too.

Borage Flower Code Indications

- When you have forgotten why you are here. Borage can help you remember and take incremental steps towards finding yourself again.
- Brings strength and courage to move forwards, to follow your heart, to face things head on and not shy away or avoid the challenges.
- Threshold crossings that require us to take action. Borage is not a passive stage. We must actively step over the threshold into the new.
- Helps us birth our hearts path, to expand our heart like a cervix dilating until our true self births itself into the world.
- To remember why you came here, your starlight sparkle mission, to remember the light within and to shine it.

- When we get stuck in a birth process, when we don't follow through when things get tough. When we lack the courage to face life head on, then invite Borage to support you and bring the courage you need.

Cherry Blossom

Nurture and Receive

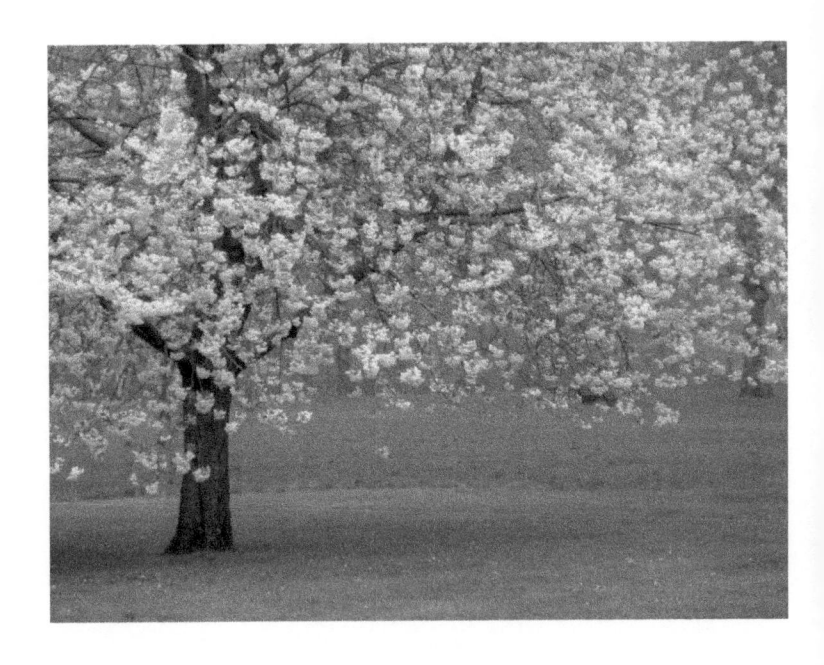

Prunus cerasus sp.

Rosaceae

Names & Etymology:

Cherry Blossom, Morello, Hawk berry, Dwarf berry, Wild cherry, Merry tree, Pie cherry, Tart cherry.

Herbal Introduction

By Pam Scott

Cherries have been domesticated from their original wild forms that were native to Europe and Western Asia. They were known as far back as 300BC when Theophrastus, the Greek father of botany spoke of them. Their popularity spread to the Romans and then into Britain where further varieties were developed. There is much confusion about these varieties. Usually the small, bushy and tart flavoured varieties, of which there were many, were classed as P. Cerasus.

Certainly, the Cerasus variety does have sour/tart flavoured cherries. The actual tree grows up to about 8 metres, which is considered smaller and bushier than the sweeter variety. Its branches and stalks are also shorter and bushier. It flowers at a later time, so isn't hit so hard with weather fluctuations, although it does need the colder weather to fruit. The fruit ripens later in the season and is a darker colour and more acidic. It is self-fertile, so isn't reliant on another to pollinate, instead suckering from the roots.

Blossoms are often the first sign of Spring, bringing hope and positivity to new projects. It is considered to be the national tree and flower of Japan, although this isn't necessarily the P. Cerasus variety. In Japan, the flowering of the Cherry Blossoms denotes a time of appreciating the beauty of nature and is known as *Hanami* – nature/flower viewing.

Cherry fruit and branches have been used for charms, spells and divination through many cultures.

Culpeper says that different tastes of the cherry, have different qualities. The tart variety is more beneficial to a hot stomach. It cuts through phlegm and gross humors. It is 'cooling in hot diseases' and increases urine and supports the bladder. Cherokees used the astringent properties of the inner root bark of P. cerasus for coughs, colds, laryngitis, fevers and wounds. An astringent decoction of the boiled fruit was beneficial for bleeding from the bowels.

This variety of cherry appears to stand on its own. This medicinal compact, self-contained, self-suckering tree that flowers and fruits at a slightly different time to others may symbolize that it is independent and all of its needs are held within. It is self-reliant.

Taking delight in the gentleness of this blossom and its gentle aroma helps you to be present and delight to the 'Hanami' within. You have everything you need at hand. From new beginnings and projects to seeing them through and bearing fruit.

Actions: Astringent, antioxidant, tryptophan, cooling, also has pain killing anthocyanins that retard the enzymes that cause tissue inflammation, so can be helpful with gout and arthritic conditions. It contains good amounts of Vitamin A and Potassium; has blood building properties; and as a low GI snack is good for diabetics.

Cherry Blossom Flower Code

Cherry Blossom is the third core flower code and the last in the Sacred Birth Portal trio. Its realm is that of new life, freshly birthed. The Cherry Blossom blooms early, heralding the imminent arrival of Spring while the world is still cool, fresh and relatively bare after Winter. It carries the associations of hope and inspiration, warmth and new life in its early tender beginnings.

Babymoon - 40 days postpartum.

Cherry Blossom relates to the time immediately after Imbolc. The roots that grew silently underground through Winter and that finally burst through to the surface of the earth at Imbolc, are now tender, soft, green shoots. Cherry Blossom at this early phase, heralds the first sign of what is to come. Soft blossoms on a skeleton tree. Energetically, this relates to the soft, vulnerable and tender newborn babe. The 40-day babymoon phase after birth is covered by Cherry Blossom. A time when a babe needs soft nurturing and round the clock tending; and the newborn mother needs to receive similar support. This is a time to be held and nurtured; softly and lovingly supported, invoking the energy of the soft, pale pink or white petals of the cherry blossom. Like the blossoms themselves, this babymoon phase doesn't last long as slowly green leaves will begin to grow on the tree, the petals will carpet the ground, and babe's senses will strengthen and grow.

Cherry Blossom is the flower code that carries the original state of feeling softly held, nurtured and gently welcomed into the world *and* within the body. It is the sensation of being held in the arms of the all loving, connected mother - nourished and comforted. Working with Cherry Blossom can awaken the latent DNA within that activates this receptive state of feeling held, nourished and joyful in the body. For some, experiencing this state for the first time may feel unfamiliar, and wounds may arise. Working with the healing herb flower codes in tandem may be required to soothe and heal through this process.

Incarnation and Awakening the Senses

Innate within the Cherry Blossom code, is the feeling of pleasure within the body and the joy of the senses awakening in an open, soft, gentle and pleasurable way. This directly affects our capacity to *receive* the world around us (via the senses) and to feel nurtured and held in the world, as well as our capacity to be fully in the body.

Cherry blossom holds the coding to incarnate gently into our bodies. The gentle creation of pleasure through the senses helps babe enter more fully into the body and arrive on the earth. The early postpartum time is where this state is naturally activated through oxytocin. Breastfeeding, plenty of skin to skin contact, co-regulation, and gentle, loving touch are all important to awaken the newborn senses in a delightful, delicious way. Equally important is gentle shielding from loud noises, excessive bright lights etc., so that the senses can become used to the new world gently, rather than be in shock or on high alert (this triggers adrenalin and stress chemistry).

Similar to birth, significant neural imprints are forming in this early phase of life, which impact and inform the way we experience the world throughout life. If our experience is not the nurturing, gentle description above, Cherry Blossom can support the reawakening of more nurturing ways of being and feeling held.

Cherry Blossom awakens our sensual nature, the senses being the gateways through which we experience the body. Awakening the senses gently is to become fully embodied. For a deeper look at the 12 senses, see Rudolf Steiner's work. When we are brought into the body in a wondrous way, there is a corresponding joy, hope and inspiration.

Nurture.

Activating the Cherry Blossom code is to work with nurturing. Some people easily birth projects, artworks, creations or businesses, but then become disappointed when they're not successful right away. Expecting instant maturity is one of the ways that we abandon our 'babies' by skipping this essential phase of *gentle nurture*. Acknowledging the vulnerability of our new creation, helps us to protect and gently nurture it so that it may continue to awaken and grow in its own timing. Birth is not the end product, rather the beginning of a long journey. Just like a babe, our new projects must be lovingly tended to each day and protected from harsh criticism. While a symphony may be written in a day, it is the practice and implementation of its seed that allows it to evolve and develop into its fullness.

Mother Baby Relationship. Postpartum Separation
Innate in the Cherry Blossom flower code is the unique and unified field of the mother-baby dynamic. At birth, the first of many subsequent natural and healthy separations between mother and babe occur. However, the energetic fields of mother and babe are intimately linked and will be for another seven years.

Awareness of the skin through gentle touch helps the babe to begin to feel the separating factor of its own boundary. But on an energetic level, the babe is still far from separate, remaining intimately connected with the mother's realm. Many people working with Cherry Blossom experience healing in the relationship with their mother, often through a deeper understanding of their own post-birth imprinting.

When postpartum bonding of mother and babe has been impacted, the awakening of the Cherry Blossom state may not have been activated. Drugs in labour, many birth interventions or complications, and separation at birth or in the days postpartum are all well documented to inhibit the hormone of bonding (oxytocin). This is intimately linked with postnatal depression and long-term impacts within the mother child relationship. Breastfeeding and days of skin to skin contact are essential first aids to begin to heal these wounds at their source. However if these too, are interrupted for whatever reason, a sense of disconnection, numbness or separation can follow throughout life. The time of Cherry Blossom blooming is brief but incredibly significant to the development of the fruit, just as the experience in the postpartum phase has a lifelong impact. It is never too late though, to begin to awaken this state, no matter how impacted your early phase in the world.

Cherry Blossom Flower Code Uses

- For newborn mothers - to come into the body fully after the experience of giving birth, to awaken nurturing qualities and healthy bonding.
- For newborn babes - to awaken the senses, arrive gently in the body and have healthy connection to being held, nurtured and to the mother.
- For many birth interventions or complications when separation of mother and baby occurred. Cherry Blossom helps to awaken the natural states that were never activated in the DNA due to these interruptions. Even decades later. Cherry Blossom can create a new imprint by showing us what it feels like to feel soft, held, nurtured, gently opened - to feel the senses awakened in beauty. Take for long periods in such cases. And work consciously with creating these sensations in your body.
- To support and nurture projects through their early phases (after the initial birth phase). To help enjoy the process of growing a project in its early phases. To remain embodied throughout the process.
- To awaken our capacity to receive love and nurturing. To open the senses to the world around us in a healthy way.
- To awaken our capacity to nurture and mother the self and our creations.
- To awaken our capacity to receive and be nurtured.

Postscript: Sacred Birth, Sacred Earth

Having worked as a midwife in the hospital system for several years, I'm incredibly aware of the downfalls inherent in our current birthing model. Even the best of midwives often must struggle to keep birth sacred within its confines. Yet to go without a midwife or experienced birthkeeper requires a depth of innerstanding and trust in the self that is not as common as one might think in the current era. Midwives and sacred birthkeepers know the birth threshold like the back of their hand – they know when to stand aside, reassure or step in as needed. They *are* the sacred space of birth, or an integral part of it.

Until we fully realise the long-term impact birth has on us, our culture will keep accepting the subtle violence and violation that is dished out as 'normal' in today's birthing systems. Each person who engages in birth imprint exploration and reclamation adds to the cultural shift. You may be the teacher of the friendly, smiling hospital caregiver who truly believes you shouldn't feel pain. Each woman who stands for the long-term effects *as well as* the short-term survival of her child, advocates for sacred birth and a change in the system. As the culture of birth changes, so will the connection we have with ourselves, others and the earth we live upon. Peace on Earth, really does begin with birth.

Resources

Flower Codes:

For flower code essences, online training and practitioners, visit www.theflowercodes.com or www.wildflowerwalker.com

Birth Imprint Exploration in various forms:

www.wildflowerwalker.com/flower-codes-training/
www.wildflowerwalker.com/bloomingmoon-sacredbirth/
www.ishasoulseededucation.com/birth-imprints/
www.birthintobeing.com.au
www.janehardwickecollings.com   (Four Seasons Journey)

Sarah Buckley's book *Gentle Birth, Gentle Mothering*, 2009, Celestial Arts. Or start here: www.sarahbuckley.com/healing-birth-healing-the-earth/

About the Authors

Pam Scott

Pam began her herbal journey in the late 1990's. She completed a 3-year Herbal Medicine Diploma course with Kim Dudley at the Hierophant in Canberra and continued her studies there for another couple of years participating in some Herbal extension lectures and a year of Homeopathy with Tim Thomas. After another 2 years at The Dorothy Hall College of Herbal Medicine, she received an Advanced Diploma of Herbal Medicine. Through this course she also studied Nutrition, Iridology, Astrology and Bach Flower Therapy. She has also spent extended periods of time over the last twenty years studying with renowned American Herbalist, Matthew Wood. In 2013 she received a Diploma in Biochemic Therapy, and still uses these Tissue Salts as an integral part of her prescription protocol.

For over 15 years, Pam was the Practitioner at Canberra's popular Health/Wholefoods shop, Mountain Creek Wholefoods where she was able to help people with a wide variety of dietary advice and many other issues and ailments.

She also worked at The Hierophant for a few years dispensing Herbal and Homeopathic Medicines. She has also studied Swedish Massage, Kinesiology, Kinergy and has a strong interest and love for Jungian Psychology after taking her own journey with a Jungian Analyst, exploring dreams and symbols for over 4 years.

She now lives on the South Coast. With such a diversity of modalities and experience, Pam can weave a wellness prescription for your well-being. www.weavingwellness.com.au

Heidi Wedd

With a history deeply embedded with plants, herbalism, homeopathy and midwifery, Heidi is passionate about reawakening and deepening our innate connection with nature. She offers a range of courses in nature connection, herbal alchemy & plant spirit communication, including the Flower Codes Training Shamanic Herbalism pathways via www.wildflowerwalker.com

Author of *Wild Flower Walker: A Pilgrimage to Nature on the Bibbulmun Track*, she writes regularly at: www.mythicliving.substack.com

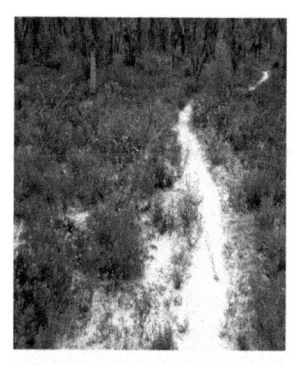

Wild Flower Walker:
A Pilgrimage to Nature on the Bibbulmun Track.

WILD FLOWER WALKER
A Pilgrimage to Nature on the Bibbulmun Track

Heidi Wedd

"Absolutely loved it. I couldn't put it down - the journey, the words, the inner knowing and learning is inspiring. It is a book I will gift to loved ones. "
J.M

She imagined the bliss of walking for weeks on end, the silence of being alone and the space to commune more deeply with nature spirits. But will the nonstop challenges of reality hinder her dream of a deeper union with nature?

This is the engaging story of a young woman solo hiking 1000km through Western Australia's wildflower filled bush. On a quest to listen more deeply to nature and despite a myriad of challenges and adventures along the way, what unfolds is a reweaving and reconnection into the very heart of nature.

Find yourself within nature's intricate tapestry as you walk the Bibbulmun track alongside her.

Available at www.wildflowerwalker.com or all your online bookstores.

Book 2

in

The Flower Codes series

coming soon!

Plant Spirit Teachings for your Soul to Blossom:

Herbal Healers